Anti-Inflar

Easy 7 Day

Recipes to Eliminate Pain

Discover a Quick 7 Day Meal Plan to Improve your Health and Eliminate the Pain of Inflammation

By: Mary Walsh

Mary Walsh

Publisher Notes

Disclaimer

This publication is intended to provide helpful and informative material. It is not intended to diagnose, treat, cure, or prevent any health problem or condition, nor is intended to replace the advice of a physician. No action should be taken solely on the contents of this book. Always consult your physician or qualified health-care professional on any matters regarding your health and before adopting any suggestions in this book or drawing inferences from it.

The author and publisher specifically disclaim all responsibility for any liability, loss or risk, personal or otherwise, which is incurred as a consequence, directly or indirectly, from the use or application of any contents of this book.

Any and all product names referenced within this book are the trademarks of their respective owners. None of these owners have sponsored, authorized, endorsed, or approved this book.

Always read all information provided by the manufacturers' product labels before using their

Mary Walsh

products. The author and publisher are not responsible for claims made by manufacturers.

Table of Contents

Mary Walsh

CHAPTER 4 - 7 Day Meal Plan for Anti Inflammatory Diet 37

CHAPTER 5 - Anti-Inflammatory Diet Breakfast Recipes ... 45

CHAPTER 6 - Anti-Inflammatory Diet Lunch Recipes 55

CHAPTER 7 - Anti-Inflammatory Diet Dinner Recipes 65

Mary Walsh

DEDICATION

This book is dedicated to Paul, for giving me an inspiration to come up with a book to help millions who are on the same arthritic condition.

Mary Walsh

Introduction

Why Anti-Inflammatory Diets?

For sure you have read or heard about a lot of diet regimen. While most of the health diets you have read of are healthy and good for the health, there is one health diet that is worth looking at. The anti-inflammatory diet is perhaps one of the most reliable diets for those suffering from arthritis and appendicitis.

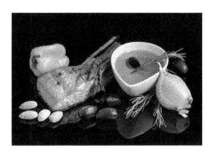

According to studies, While each diets target health goals, everything seem to root from a general idea of battling diseases and keeping the systems of the body function at its best. Anti-inflammatory diets target frequent inflammation in the body that leads to serious health disorders. Eating the right foods eases inflammation and promotes better function of the body organs.

The most extreme diet I have ever known is the anti-inflammatory diet (presented in this book in the simplest manner understandable by many). Even when the diet is not fully implemented, it still instills good transformation in the body that is beneficial for your health.

Small changes like removing the use of white flour in your household, or the use of white sugar and non-organic meat products are a great way to start. Alternatively, consumption of whole wheat, organic fruits and vegetables, molasses and organically produced meats are evident to enhance one's health.

These small changes in the household do not have to happen overnight. Taking small steps each day are gradual changed that eventually leads the whole family to healthier eating habits. In some cases, abrupt changes in the household are done if one of the members of the family has gotten ill.

As many doctors have pointed out, prevention is better than cure. Changing to a healthier eating habit prevents illnesses that are detrimental and allows each member of the family to have a better resistance to common illnesses. This diet has a true potential to cleanse the body from toxins and eliminate the possibilities of inflammation in the body.

The Silent Killer

Inflammation is a silent killer as proven by many instances of health cases throughout the world. Arthritis and Appendicitis involve inflammation including heart diseases and even the ever known Alzheimer's disease.

The American diet alone proves to include far too many omega-6 fatty acids, which are found in many processed foods and even food you find in fast food chains. The diet alone contains very few omega-3 fatty acids, which are commonly found in cold water fish. When there is an imbalance of this kind, there is a higher chance for inflammation in the body, which can be very detrimental to health.

CHAPTER 1
-
Anti-Inflammatory Diet Overview

An anti-inflammatory diet is a diet plan that seeks to reduce inflammation in the body while at the same time giving a good source of energy and sufficient vitamins and minerals as well as healthy fatty acids, protective phytonutrients and dietary fibers.

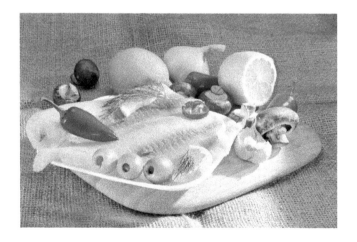

Top 10 Anti-Inflammatory Foods

Wild Alaskan Salmon

Salmon is a very good source of omega-3, which makes it a good addition to anti-inflammatory diet. If fish does not appeal to you, an alternative would be to add a high quality fish supplement to your diet plan.

Kelp

Kelp is very high in fiber. This brown algae is a great help to regulate liver and lung cancer cells, relieves inflammation. Kelp, being high in antioxidants, is also good to fight tumor. Some other good sources of antioxidants are kombu, wakame, and arame.

Olive Oil

Olive oil has been said to be the secret of Mediterranean culture for a longer life. A lot of health benefits can be derived from it such as lessening the dangers of asthma attacks, arthritis, and it even protects the heart and blood vessels from inflammation that may cause serious health issues.

Cruciferous Vegetables

Vegetables from the cruciferous family such Brussels sprouts, broccoli, cauliflower, and kale are rich in anti-oxidants. These vegetables have the ability to detoxify the body of harmful toxins.

Blueberries

Blueberries are a good source of dietary fibers and vitamin c. It has the ability to reduce inflammation and prevent premature brain aging. Blueberries are also known to prevent various diseases like dementia and cancer. Beware of pesticides, choose organic berries.

Turmeric

Tumeric, a potent Asian herb is rich in curcumin, a natural anti-inflammatory compound. Curcumin is usually found in many curry blends. Tumeric has a pain relieving effect which resembles over the counter pain reliever drugs without the side effects.

Ginger

Ginger provides several health benefits. Ginger naturally assists in the reduction of inflammation and regulates blood sugar well. Consider adding ginger tea to your daily diet.

Garlic
Garlic has unique sulfur compounds known as 1,2-DT (1,2-vinyldithiin), which makes garlic a good addition to anti-inflammatory diet. These sulfuric compounds aids in the reduction of inflammation manage glucose and boost the body's immune system to fight infection.

Green Tea
Green tea has flavonoids, which help reduce inflammation. It also has the ability to reduce the dangers of cancer.

Sweet Potato
Sweet potato is a good source of fiber, complex carbs, beta-carotene, vitamin b6, vitamin c, and manganese.

Top 10 Inflammatory Foods

These foods have actually been linked to weight problems, increased dangers of various diseases, as well as death in many cases.

Sugar

Sugar is everywhere. Try and limit processed foods, desserts, and snacks with excess sugar. Opt for fruit instead.

Typical Food Cooking Oils

Oils from safflower, soya, corn, sunflower, and cottonseed. These oils promote irritation and are made with more affordable active ingredients.

Trans Fats

Trans fats raise bad cholesterol levels, promote swelling, obesity and resistance to blood insulin. They are found in fried foods, convenience meals, commercially baked products, such as peanut butter and items readied with partly hydrogenated oil, margarine, and vegetable oil.

Dairy Products

While kefir and other yogurts are acceptable, dairy products are hard on the body. Milk is a usual allergen that can activate swelling, tummy problems, skin breakouts, hives, and even breathing problems.

Feedlot-Raised Meat

Animals which are fed with grains like soy and corn have high swelling. They additionally gain excess fat deposits and are infused with hormones and prescription antibiotics. Alternatively, go for organic, free-range meats, which have actually been fed 100% natural diets.

Red and Processed Meat

Red meat has a molecule that human beings do not normally produce called Neu5GC. Your body establishes antibodies which may trigger constant inflammatory responses once you ingest this substance. Lessen red meat usage and replace with fowl, fish, and eat cuts of red meat, once in a week's time at most.

Liquor

Regular intake of liquor causes irritation and inflammation to various body organs, which could bring about cancer cells.

Refined Grains

Refined products have no fiber and have a higher glycemic index. You can find them commonly in white flour, white rice, white bread, and pasta... Intake of minimally processed grains is advisable.

Synthetic Food Additives

Aspartame and MSG are two common food additives that can activate inflammation and irritation responses. It is best to leave these synthetic additives completely out from the diet plan.

Foods that trigger allergies you are not aware of

Are you often tired? Are you experiencing frequent migraines? In some cases, you might develop an allergy to meals and not even recognize it. Take a few foods out to find out exactly how you feel. And then, slowly incorporate them back to your diet to see which of the foods give you these symptoms.

Mary Walsh

CHAPTER 2
-
Inflammation Health Information

Inflammation: The Root Cause of All Disease?

What is inflammation?

Inflammation: A physical disorder where part of the physical body becomes reddened, swollen, hot, and often painful, specifically as a reaction to injury or infection.

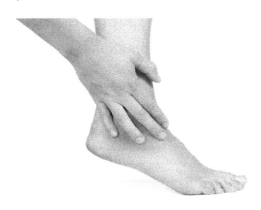

We all know when something is inflamed because it is visible to the eye. But what about inflammation that takes place inside our body?

Internal inflammation could take place for a host of reasons: high temperatures when cooking meals, consuming refined foods, sweets, trans fats, and so on. A high degree of irritation within the body could induce many health issues.

What is a simple way to fight this? Eat even more anti-inflammatory meals, and eliminate the inflammatory ones.

What is an anti-inflammatory food?

You can distinguish healthy and whole foods from processed and unhealthy foods. However some of us may not see the effects it could bring inside our body. More often than not, it is too late to realize that we have internal inflammation.

More often than not, many diseases are a reflection of what we eat. As an example, diseases like diabetes, Polycystic Ovarian Syndrome (PCOS), excess weight, heart disease and others are results of inflammation from many foods causing inflammation.

Top Warning Sign of Persistent Inflammation

1. The quickest method to know if your body—and arteries—may be ablaze is to determine your waistline. A circumference over 35 inches for a lady or 40 inches for a guy indicates you could be at risk for a range of dangerous diseases associated with persistent inflammation, an indication even if your weight shows normal.

2. Too much visceral fat is far different from other fat in the body. Abdominal fat cells are a lot more biologically energetic in comparison to subcutaneous fatty tissue cells; releasing many bodily hormones and cytokines [chemical messengers associated with immune system and inflamed feedbacks].

3. There is also a hereditary component to both chronic inflammation and weight problems—it's not merely an unhealthy way of living that brings about these problems.

4. A large tummy (big belly) is also the leading sign of metabolic disorder. Fifty million Americans, several of whom are undiagnosed, suffer from this hazardous condition.

If you have three or more of the following disorders, you have metabolic syndrome:

- A huge midsection, usually called "an apple form."
- High triglycerides: a blood fat level over 150 mg/dL.
- Low HDL (much less than 50 mg/dL for women and less than 40 mg/dL for men). HDL is the good cholesterol that maintains balance in the heart and brain.
- High blood pressure: 130/85 mmHg or greater (or if you're on bp meds).
- High fasting blood glucose: 100 mg/dL or over (or if you're on meds to cope with higher blood sugar).

CHAPTER 3
-
Anti-inflammatory Dietary Tips

Anti-Inflammatory Diet Starts With Healthy Eating

Eating healthy is not about meticulous nutrition philosophies, staying unrealistically slim, or denying yourself of the foods you love.

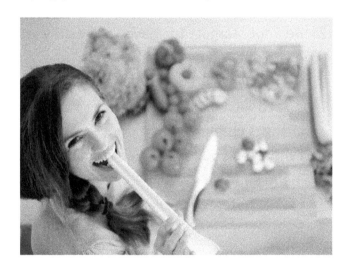

Instead, it's about really feeling great, having additional electricity, maintaining your state of mind, and remaining to be as healthy and balanced as possible—all of which could be attained by discovering some nourishment fundamentals and using them in such a way that works for you.

You can increase your array of healthy meal options, and find out ways to plan in advance to make and keep a delicious, healthy, and balanced diet regimen.

Some small tips to succeed

1. Simplify your approach to diet.
2. Do not target to have a healthy diet overnight.
3. Small changes that are done every day are turned into habits, which make succeeding changes easier.
4. Every step you take to boost your diet plan in the end.
5. Make water and exercise as among the food groups in your diet

Tips to eating with moderation

1. For the majority of us, moderation or balance means consuming much less in

comparison to we do now. But it does not suggest doing away with the meals you like.

2. Moderate eating may mean eating bacon for a morning meal once a week can be considered moderation if you follow it with a healthy and balanced lunch time and dinner—however, not if you follow it with a box of donuts and a sausage pizza.

3. Do not to think of particular meals as a taboo. When you disallow particular meals or food groups, it is 100% natural to desire those meals a lot more, and then feel like a failure if you succumb to lure.

4. Assume smaller sized portions. Serving sizes have ballooned just recently, particularly in bistros. When dining out, decide on a starter instead of an entree, divide a meal with a good friend, and don't attempt to buy supersized meals or beverages.

5. If you don't really feel completely satisfied at the end of a meal, try including more leafed green veggies or settling the dish with fresh fruit.

Tips to be conscious of what you eat and how you eat

1. Eat with others whenever feasible. Eating with other people has numerous social and emotional advantages—particularly for youngsters—and permits you to design healthy eating behaviors.
2. It is advisable to take your time to munch your meals, and take pleasure in the nourishments you are going to receive.
3. Pay attention to your body. Ask yourself if you are actually famished, or have a glass of water to see if you are thirsty instead of starving.
4. Consume breakfast, and consume smaller sized meals throughout the day.
5. Avoid eating at night. Try to consume dinner previously in the day, and then fast for 14-16 hrs until the morning meal the following day.

Eat colorful fruits and vegetables

Some great choices include:

- For your greens, choose bright dark and green like lettuce, kale, mustard greens, broccoli, and cabbage. These choices are rich with vitamins A, C, E, and K, calcium, iron, magnesium, zinc, and potassium
- Add sweet vegetables to your daily meal. Sweet vegetable choices include squash, sweet potatoes, yams, carrots, beets, and corn. Adding these healthy sweets reduces your cravings for other unhealthy items.
- Don't forget your fruits, a good source of antioxidants and other nutrients such as vitamins and fiber. Eat more of the healthy carbs and whole grains

Healthy carbs vs. unhealthy carbs

Healthy carbs or good carbs are carbohydrates coming from beans, whole grains, vegetables, and fruits. Healthy carbs take time to be digested, which helps you feel full for a longer period, which helps stabilize the blood sugar and insulin levels.

Unhealthy carbs or bad carbs are carbohydrates coming from whiter flour, white rice, and refined sugar. These food products have gone through thorough processes. The nutrients have been stripped away from these food products throughout the process. Unhealthy carbs are easy to digest and can spike up insulin and blood sugar levels.

Eat healthy fats & stay away from unhealthy fats

Great addition to healthy diet

1. Monounsaturated fats. Sources are plant oils extracted from canola, peanut, and olives. Oils extracted from avocados, nuts (almonds, hazelnuts, and pecans), and seeds (pumpkin, sesame) are also good sources.

2. Polyunsaturated fats. This includes Omega-6 and Omega-3 fatty acids. Sources are fatty fish like salmon, mackerel, herring, sardines, and anchovies. Other sources include unheated sunflower, flaxseed oils, soybean, corn, and walnuts.

Remove from your diet

1. Saturated fats are found in animal sources, which include whole milk dairy products.
2. Trans fats found in vegetable shortenings. Examples are margarines, candies, crackers, cookies, fried foods, snack foods, baked goods, and other processed foods (usually made from not fully hydrogenated vegetable oils).

Guidelines to include protein in your healthy diet

1. Trying out various protein sources will open new alternatives for healthier meals. Other protein sources include soy, grains, tofu, nuts, greens, and seeds.
2. Limit your consumption of protein. Instead of eating more of the protein foods, focus on having equal portions of foods from protein, whole grains, and vegetables.
3. Focus on getting proteins from quality sources like fresh fish, poultry, tofu, eggs, beans, and even nuts. When opting to get protein from meat, choose meats from safe sources.

For stronger bones: consume more foods rich in calcium

Great sources for calcium needs

1. Dairy: Dairy products like milk, cheese and yogurt are very rich in calcium. They are even in a structure that the body can easily digest and absorb.

2. Vegetables and greens: Leafy vegetables are great sources of calcium. Like mustard greens, turnip greens, collard greens, celery, broccoli, fennel, cabbage, green beans, Brussels sprouts, romaine lettuce, crimini mushrooms, and kale are great additions to your daily meals to get the needed calcium for the body.

3. Beans: Try pinto beans, black beans, kidney beans, baked beans, white beans, or black-eyed peas; they are all rich in calcium.

Tips to help you lessen sugar intake

1. Stay away from those sugary drinks. Try drinking fresh and sparkling water. It has more nutrients than a 12-oz soda that has about 10 tsp of sugar, more than what the

body needs. It is also recommended to drink water with lemon or a splash of fruit juice.

2. Put the sugar yourself, it is more likely to control sugar if you are the one to sweeten your food. Purchase the foods that are unsweetened, like iced tea, plain yogurt, or unflavored oatmeal, and you should be the one to add sweetener or a fruit if you prefer.

3. Naturally-sweetened foods are great in sugar consumption control. Fruit, peppers, or natural peanut butter are better than candy or cookies; they are more likely to have the right amount of sugar to satisfy that sweet tooth.

Guides in lessening salt intake

1. Processed or pre-packaged foods have high sodium content because salt is usually used for preservation. Canned soups or frozen dinners have high salt content that you may even not be aware of, or taste for that matter.

2. When eating out, be more careful because most foods that they serve in restaurants and fast food establishments have huge amount of sodium. You can ask for a meal without salt, or choose among the low-sodium dishes they offer. As well as most sauce and gravy, they are rich in salt, so request for it to be on a separate side dish.

3. You should always choose fresh or frozen greens, not the canned or preserved vegetables. Cut the consumption of those salty snacks such as nuts, pretzels, and potato chips as well. Always check the product labels when you go to the grocery. Opt for the reduce-sodium items. Lastly, a slow pace in salt reduction will help your diet, it will help your taste palettes to adjust to the new taste and diet plan.

CHAPTER 4
-
7 Day Meal Plan for Anti Inflammatory Diet

Inflammation can be controlled through our food intake. Foods with anti-inflammatory properties have been proven effective. You can manage that rheumatoid arthritis with these full week meal plan. Savor tasty dishes with the ease of avoiding pain caused by inflammations.

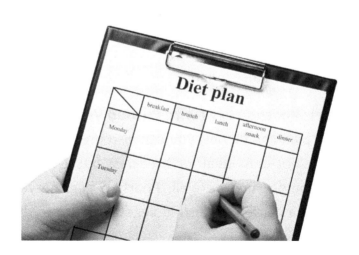

Day One

Breakfast: Cherry Quinoa Porridge

A traditional porridge is an ideal meal for your breakfast. Try using the super-grain: quinoa on this hearty meal, and you'll get more healthy benefits. In addition, when you put dried or fresh tart cherries, with its substantial amount of anthocyanin, it will surely drive inflammations away. A great way to start your day is a healthy and tasty breakfast.

Lunch: Quick-and-Easy Pumpkin Soup

Beta-cryptoxanthin is a powerful substance for anti-inflammatory, and pumpkins have a lot of it. Prepare and cooked with ginger, and you'll have the ideal recipe for arthritis. Savor this tasty recipe and prevent those inflammation issues.

Dinner: Poached Eggs with Curried Vegetables

When planning dinner, you can also prepare eggs. They're not only ideal for breakfast but great for meals before bed as well. Poached eggs served lying on a garden of curried vegetables are to die for.

Day Two

Breakfast: Raspberry Green Tea Smoothie

Rushing to go to work or not, you need a great breakfast to satisfy the huger. This smoothie recipe is a fantastic drink to give you all that.

Lunch: Kipper's Salad

It is also known as smoked herring; kippers also have a substantial amount of Omega-3. This fatty acid is very helpful in making inflammation minimal. A great alternative if you can't find tuna, kippers are very tasty and delicious, especially if prepared with a special salad.

Dinner: Weeknight Turkey Chili

Nothing beats chili when you are cold. With this easy to prepare recipe, you can say good bye to those cold nights. This dish is so tasty and so healthy; it has nutrients that will reduce the issues of your Arthritis.

Day Three

Breakfast: Gingerbread Oatmeal

If you are having trouble with joint inflammation, arthritis, or any other joint problems, but you need to go to work early in the morning, you need a hearty breakfast. Gingerbread oatmeal is a magical way to start your day.

Lunch: Roasted Chicken Wraps

Do you have some leftovers of roasted chicken you ordered last night? Make this easy treat to pack those tummy for lunch. It's not just tasty but healthy as well.

Dinner: Brazil Nut-Crusted Tilapia with Sautéed Kale

Selenium is a mineral that helps anyone to minimize any arthritis symptoms and arthritis itself. Brazil nuts together with tilapia are packed with selenium.

Day Four

Breakfast: Ginger Apple Muffins

Bread and butter is not enough, especially if you have a tendency of joints inflammation. Start your day well and right with this quick-and-easy muffins.

Lunch: Persimmon and Pear Salad

In preparing a veggie salad be sure to set aside your dressing at first so not to wilt the freshness of your greens. If you want to take this recipe to work, place the mix and the dressing on separate containers.

Dinner: Red Pepper and Turkey Pasta

It is very usual when we speak of pasta, we think of tomato sauce and spaghetti. Instead of the tomato-based pasta, why not try a twist on your sauce? Consider this recipe that uses red peppers, which are full of vitamin C and beta-carotene.

Day Five

Breakfast: Buckwheat and Quinoa Granola

For an energizing breakfast, try this wheat-free granola topped with almond milk. You can also use soy yogurt if you prefer.

Lunch: Roasted Sweet Potato Soup

If you have no time to heat your food, this is a great make-ahead soup that freezes beautifully.

Dinner: Steamed Salmon with Lemon Scented Zucchini

Steaming is a great way to cook and lock in the flavors, moisture, vitamins, and minerals of your favorite protein. With this recipe, you'll enjoy the taste of salmon with all its glorious flavors.

Day Six

Breakfast: Spinach and Mushroom Frittata

Frittatas are like omelets and quiches; it can provide you with such tasty choices ingredients on the backdrop. In this recipe, we'll use the healthy and nutritious combination of mushrooms and spinach, a very tasty and hearty breakfast.

Lunch: Smoked Trout Tartine

With this recipe and a side of soup, it will surely satisfy your lunchtime. This famous Parisian dish is often served like an open-faced sandwich that will make your tummy ask for more.

Dinner: Sweet Potato and Black Bean Burgers with Lime Mayonnaise

You might give up that usual fast food beef burger once you taste this fantastic burger. High in vitamin C, beta-carotene and delicious, what more can you ask for a burger well in fact it's all here.

Day Seven

Breakfast: Gluten Free Strawberry Crepes
Most of us think that crepes are difficult to cook or make. We usually have the thought that this is only for special occasions. In fact, it is very easy to prepare and very good for breakfast.

Lunch: Lentil and Garbanzo Soup
This great soup freezes beautifully, so you can prepare it ahead of time. It even tastes better the next day. Just remember to thaw it first just enough to reheat in the microwave when the lunch bell rings.

Dinner: Quinoa and Turkey Stuffed Peppers
This is a very 1950's classic dish: the stuffed peppers. Quinoa is one of the world's most powerful super-foods, and with turkey you will definitely heighten the flavor. You can also go for the red, yellow, or orange peppers for a sweeter taste.

Mary Walsh

CHAPTER 5
-
Anti-Inflammatory Diet Breakfast Recipes

In this chapter, you will find healthy, easy to prepare breakfast recipes to fight inflammation.

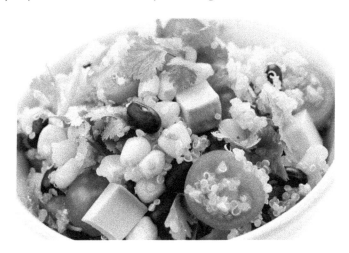

Cherry Quinoa Porridge

Ingredients
- 1 cup of water
- 1/2 cup of dry quinoa
- 1/2 cup of dried unsweetened cherries
- 1/2 tsp. vanilla extract

- 1/4 tsp. ground cinnamon
- 1 tbsp. honey (optional)

Preparations

1. Stir all ingredients except honey in a medium-sized saucepan.
2. Over a medium heat, bring it to a boil
3. Gradual stirring to avoid burning.
4. Lower the heat.
5. Cover and simmer for 15 minutes.
6. Done when quinoa is tender and all the water is absorbed.
7. Put in cup and drizzle with honey.
8. Enjoy your healthy breakfast.

Raspberry Green Tea Smoothie

Ingredients

- 1½ cups of chilled green tea
- 2 cups of unsweetened raspberries (frozen)
- 1 banana
- 1 tbsp. of honey
- ¼ cup of protein powder

Preparations

1. With your blender, put in all the ingredients and blend.

2. Place in your favorite cup and enjoy.

Gingerbread Oatmeal

Ingredients
- 1 cup of water
- ½ cup of old-fashioned oats
- ¼ cup unsweetened cherries/cranberries (dried)
- 1 tsp of ground ginger
- ½ tsp of ground cinnamon
- ¼ tsp of ground nutmeg
- 1 tbsp. of flaxseeds
- 1 tbsp. of molasses

Preparations
1. In a small saucepan, mix all water, oats, cranberries or cherries, cinnamon, and nutmeg.
2. Turn heat on medium-high.
3. Bring the mix to a boil.
4. Reduce heat and let it simmer.
5. Let the water be reduced or slightly absorbed, usually it takes 5 minutes.
6. Mix in flaxseeds.
7. Let it stand for about 5 minutes, covered.

8. Drizzled it with molasses and serve.

Ginger Apple Muffins

Ingredients
- 2 cups of all-purpose flour
- ⅔ cup of sugar or sugar-substitute granules
- 1 tbsp. of baking powder
- ½ tsp. of salt
- 1 tsp. ground cinnamon
- 1 tsp. of ground ginger
- ¾ cup of unsweetened almond milk
- 1 cup of shredded apple
- ½ cup of ripe and mashed banana
- 1 tbsp. of apple cider vinegar
- ½ cup of crystallized ginger (finely chopped)

Preparations
1. Prepare your oven by preheating it on 400°F.
2. You can use paper liners, or if you are using muffin pan, grease it lightly.
3. In a medium-sized bowl, blend in together flour, sugar, baking powder, salt, cinnamon and ginger.

4. Set aside and mix milk, apple, banana, and vinegar in a large bowl

5. Then mix in the flour mixture until blended well.

6. Fill your muffin cups in just about ⅔ full.

7. Start baking for about 15 to 20 minutes

8. Insert toothpick in the center, if it comes out clean, then you're done.

9. Serve with your favorite juice and have a healthy day.

Buckwheat and Quinoa Granola

Ingredients

- 3 tbsp. of honey
- 3 tbsp. of liquid coconut oil
- 1 tsp. of vanilla extract
- ¼ tsp. of ground cinnamon
- ¼ tsp. of ground ginger
- 1 cup of buckwheat oats
- 1 cup of cooked quinoa
- ½ cup of old-fashioned oats
- ½ cup of unsweetened cranberries (dried)

Preparations

1. Prepare oven with a 325°F temp.

2. Prepare baking sheet with light grease, or ready your silicon baking mat.
3. Mix your honey, coconut oil, vanilla extract, cinnamon, and ground ginger in a small bowl.
4. Set aside first.
5. Then, mix buckwheat, quinoa, and oats in a large bowl.
6. Blend in your honey mixture thoroughly.
7. In prepared pan, spread the mixture evenly to be baked evenly as well.
8. Bake it in your oven preheated with 325°F.
9. When grains start to brown, usually takes 40 to 45 minutes, remove and mix in cranberries.
10. Make sure to cool it completely before placing in airtight storage.

Spinach and Mushroom Frittata

Ingredients
- 1 lb. of button mushrooms (sliced)
- 1 large onion (chopped)
- 1 tbsp. of fresh garlic (chopped)
- 1 lb. of fresh spinach
- ¼ cup of water

- 6 large egg whites
- 4 large eggs
- 5 oz. of firm tofu
- ½ tsp. of ground turmeric
- ½ tsp. of kosher salt
- ½ tsp. of freshly cracked black pepper

Preparations

1. Prepare and preheat your oven to 350°F.
2. On a lightly greased sauté pan and medium-high heat, sauté your mushrooms until golden brown.
3. Add in your onion, cook it until tender, usually takes about 3 minutes.
4. Put in garlic and cook for about 30 seconds
5. Put in spinach and add water
6. Cover it and cook for 2 minutes, until the spinach is wilted.
7. Uncover and let the liquid evaporate.
8. In a blender, puree the egg whites, tofu, eggs, salt, pepper, and turmeric until smooth.
9. Pour mixture gently on your spinach when excess liquid is gone.
10. Put pan in oven and bake.

11. Remove from oven for about 25 to 30 minutes, eggs will set in the center.
12. Let it stand for 10 minutes.
13. Cut and serve in wedges.

Gluten Free Strawberry Crepes

Ingredients

- 6 cups of strawberries (sliced)
- 2 tbsp. of sugar or honey
- 4 large eggs
- 1 cup of unsweetened almond milk
- 2 tbsp. of light olive oil
- 1 tsp. of vanilla extract
- 1 tbsp. of light brown sugar
- ⅛ tsp. of salt
- ¾ cup gluten free flour (baking mix)

Preparations

1. Mix your strawberries and sugar in a clean container.
2. Let it stand for 30 minutes in a room temperature.
3. Whisk in eggs, milk, olive oil, vanilla, sugar, light sugar, and salt in a medium-size bowl until well-combined.

4. Blend in the flour and mix it well.
5. Heat a non-stick crepe pan, about 8 to 9 inch in diameter.
6. Pour about ¼ cup of the batter on pan.
7. Swirl and to completely coat the non-stick pan.
8. Flip your crepe when it starts to turn brown to cook the other side. This usually takes 30 to 40 seconds.
9. The other side usually takes 10 seconds.
10. Be watchful to avoid burnt crepes.
11. Place it on a serving plate.
12. Spoon an about ½ cup of the strawberry mix and place it on the middle of the crepe.
13. Fold the crepe into a semicircle to cover the strawberries.
14. Drizzle the juices from your strawberry mixture for more flavors.
15. Serve and enjoy.

Mary Walsh

CHAPTER 6
-
Anti-Inflammatory Diet Lunch Recipes

Find lunch recipes that are really easy to prepare and a great combination of ingredients to fight inflammation.

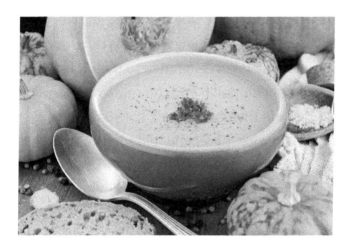

Quick-and-Easy Pumpkin Soup

Ingredients
- 1 cup of onion (chopped)
- 1 1-inch piece gingerroot, (peeled and minced)
- 1 clove of garlic (minced)

- 6 cups vegetable stock, divided
- 4 cups of pumpkin puree
- 1 tsp. of salt
- ½ tsp. of fresh thyme (chopped)
- ½ cup of half-and-half
- 1 tsp. of fresh parsley (chopped)

Preparations

1. Over a medium-high heat, prepare your large soup pot
2. Put and cook your onions, garlic, ginger, and half-cup of vegetable stock.
3. Usually takes 5 minutes to be tender.
4. Put in pumpkin and the remaining stock.
5. Mix in thyme and cook for 30 minutes.
6. Use your handheld blender to puree the mixture to turn it into a smooth and aromatic soup.
7. Remove and turn-of the heat
8. Stir and mix in your half-and-half.
9. Serve and sprinkle your soup with chopped parsley for a more aromatic and delicious delight.

Kippers Salad

Ingredients

- ½ cup of reduced fat mayonnaise
- 1 small onion (finely chopped)
- 1 celery stalk (finely chopped)
- 1 tbsp of fresh parsley (chopped)
- 1 tsp of lemon juice
- 1 clove garlic (minced)
- ⅛ tsp of salt
- ⅛ tsp of ground black pepper
- 1 (6-ounce) can of kippers (drained)

Preparations

1. Mix your ingredients except the kippers in a medium-sized bowl.
2. Stir and toss until well incorporated.
3. Gently toss in your flaked kippers.
4. Refrigerate first until you are ready to serve it.
5. Enjoy with a hearty drink.

Roasted Chicken Wraps

Ingredients

- ½ cup of reduced fat mayonnaise
- 2 tbsp of pickle juice
- 1 tsp freshly cracked black pepper
- 1½ cups of shredded red cabbage
- 1 tbsp of apple cider vinegar
- ¼ tsp of kosher salt
- ¼ tsp of cayenne pepper
- 1 cooled deli-roasted chicken
- 6 whole wheat or mixed grain flatbreads

Preparations

1. In a large bowl, mix and combine the pickle juice, mayonnaise, and pepper.
2. Set aside and refrigerate.
3. Toss and combine cabbage, vinegar, salt, and cayenne pepper in a medium-sized bowl.
4. Set aside.
5. Meanwhile, discard the skin and bones of the roasted chicken.
6. Shred the chicken into bite-sized pieces.
7. Mix in the chicken with your mayonnaise mixture.
8. Stir it thoroughly, to blend mixture with chicken.

9. Evenly spread the chicken and cabbage mixture on your flatbread slices.
10. Roll the bread to secure stuffing.
11. Serve and enjoy.

Persimmon and Pear Salad

Ingredients

- 1 tsp. of whole grain mustard
- 2 tbsp. of fresh lemon juice
- 3 tbsp. of extra virgin olive oil
- 1 shallot (minced)
- 1 tsp. of garlic (minced)
- 1 ripe persimmon (sliced)
- 1 ripe red pear (sliced)
- ½ cup pecans (toasted and chopped)
- 6 cups of baby spinach

Preparations

1. Mix and whisk mustard, lemon juice, olive oil, shallots, and garlic in a large salad bowl.
2. Put in your persimmons.
3. Add pear, pecans, and spinach.
4. Toss well, to evenly coat ingredients with the mixture.
5. Serve it immediately.

Mary Walsh

Roasted Sweet Potato Soup

Ingredients
- 2½ lbs. of sweet potatoes
- 1 tbsp. of extra virgin olive oil
- ¼ tsp. of kosher salt
- ½ tsp. of freshly cracked pepper
- 1½ cups of thinly sliced leeks or onions
- 1 1-inch piece of ginger (peeled and minced)
- 1 tsp. garlic (minced)
- ½ cup of dry white wine
- 1 tsp of fresh thyme leaves (chopped)
- 5 cups of vegetable broth
- 2 cups of orange juice

Preparations
1. First, prepare your oven, preheated to about 400ºF.
2. Cut your peeled sweet potatoes into pieces about an inch small.
3. Place the pieces of potatoes on your baking sheet.
4. Toss in your olive oil, salt, and pepper evenly to your potatoes.
5. Roast in your oven about 45 to 50 minutes.

6. With occasional tossing, cook it until tender and well-browned.
7. Spray your large soup pot with cooking spray evenly.
8. Over a medium-high heat, cook your onions until wilted and tender, usually takes about 8 minutes.
9. Add and stir in garlic and ginger.
10. Cook for about 1 minute.
11. Pour in wine and bring to a boil.
12. Before adding broth, let the wine evaporate first.
13. Stir in the thyme and sweet potatoes.
14. Bring to a boil, reduce the heat, and let it simmer for 20 minutes.
15. When all vegetables are tender, you can now carefully puree it per batch. Use a hand-held blender for better results.
16. Reheat before serving the soup for optimal taste.

Smoked Trout Tartine

Ingredients

Mary Walsh

1. 2 tbsp. of freshly squeezed lemon juice
2. 1 tbsp. of extra virgin olive oil
3. 1 teaspoon Dijon mustard
4. Pinch of sugar
5. ¾ lb. smoked trout in bite-size pieces
6. 2 tbsp. of capers, rinsed and drained
7. ½ cup of roasted red peppers (diced)
8. 1 stalk of celery (finely chopped)
9. 2 tbsp. of onions (minced)
10. 1 tsp. of chopped fresh dill or ½ teaspoon dried dill
11. ½ (15-ounce) can cannellini beans (white kidney beans), drained and rinsed
12. 4 large, ½-inch-thick slices of crusty whole grain bread, toasted
13. dill sprigs for garnish

Preparations

1. Whisk lemon juice, olive oil, mustard and sugar in a large bowl.
2. Mix in the rest of ingredients except for the bread.
3. Toss and combine thoroughly.
4. Spoon your trout mixture into your bread evenly.

5. Garnish with the dill sprigs and serve.
6. Enjoy your lunch.

Lentil and Garbanzo Soup

Ingredients
- 2 onions, chopped
- 1 cup chopped celery
- 1 cup diced carrots
- 2 teaspoons grated fresh ginger
- 1 teaspoon minced garlic
- 1 teaspoon garam masala
- 1 teaspoon turmeric
- ½ teaspoon ground cumin
- ¼ teaspoon ground cayenne pepper
- 6 cups vegetable broth or stock
- 1 cup lentils
- 2 (15-ounce) cans garbanzo beans, rinsed and drained
- 1 (14.5-ounce) can petite diced tomatoes, undrained

Preparations
1. Set stove to medium-high heat.
2. Place your large soup pot and spray it with cooking spray.

3. For about 3 to 4 minutes, sauté the onions until tender.

4. Put in carrots and celery.

5. Cook for about 5 minutes.

6. Mix in garlic, ginger, turmeric, and garam masala.

7. Cook for about 30 seconds, then pour in your broth.

8. Put the remaining ingredients.

9. Cook the lentils until tender, usually takes about 90 minutes.

10. For a thicker and creamier soup, you can puree half of the soup, and then put it back.

CHAPTER 7
-
Anti-Inflammatory Diet Dinner Recipes

Dinner Recipes that everyone will adore; these recipes are easy to prepare and really good for the body to fight inflammation.

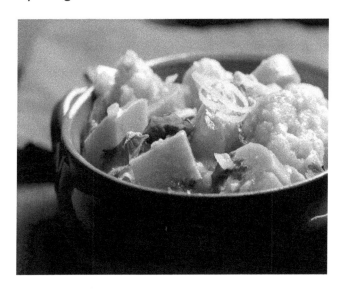

Poached Eggs with Curried Vegetables

Ingredients
- 2 tsp. of extra virgin olive oil

Mary Walsh

- 1 large onion (chopped)
- 2 cloves of garlic (minced)
- 1 tbsp. yellow curry powder
- ½ lb. of button mushrooms (sliced)
- 2 medium zucchinis (diced)
- 1 (14-ounce can) chickpeas (drained)
- 1 cup water
- ⅛ tsp of red pepper (crushed and optional)
- ½ tsp of white vinegar
- 4 large eggs

Preparations

1. Grease lightly your large nonstick skillet over medium-high heat.
2. Sauté the onions for about 4 to 5 minutes until tender.
3. Put and cook your garlic for about 30 seconds.
4. Mix in curry powder.
5. Cook for about 2 minutes until very aromatic.
6. Put the mushrooms until excess liquid is released.
7. Put your chickpeas, zucchini, and red pepper.

8. Pour in water and bring it to a boil.
9. Cover and lower heat, let it simmer.
10. Let your veggies be tender.
11. While waiting for tenderization, boil a large saucepan with about 3 inches of water.
12. For poached eggs, lower the heat and add vinegar.
13. Simmer and maintain low heat.
14. Crack eggs, and let it slip gently into the water.
15. Make it sure the eggs are close to the surface as much as possible.
16. Simmer until desired degree of doneness.
17. Retrieve egg with slotted spoon.
18. Serve your veggies with the pouched egg on top.

Weeknight Turkey Chili

Ingredients
- Vegetable cooking spray
- 1 large onion (chopped)
- 1 tbsp. garlic (minced)
- 1½ lbs. ground turkey
- 2 cups of water
- 1 (28-ounce) can canned crushed tomatoes

- 2 tsp. turmeric
- 1 tsp. smoked paprika
- 1 tsp. dried oregano
- 1 tsp. ground cumin
- 1 tsp. hot sauce
- 1 (16-ounce) can canned kidney beans, drained and rinsed

Preparations

1. Spray your large soup pot with cooking spray evenly.
2. About 5 minutes, cook onions until it starts to brown and get tender.
3. Add and cook garlic for about 30 seconds.
4. Put the turkey and stir occasionally until cooked.
5. Pour in water, and add remaining ingredients.
6. Bring to a boil.
7. Lower the heat and let it simmer.
8. Leave it uncovered for 30 to 45 minutes.
9. Serve and enjoy your dinner.

Brazil Nut-Crusted Tilapia with Sautéed Kale

Ingredients

- ¼ cup roasted Brazil nuts
- ½ cup fresh bread crumbs
- 2 tablespoons grated Parmesan cheese
- ¼ cup whole grain mustard
- 1½ pounds tilapia fillets
- Vegetable cooking spray
- 1 tablespoon sesame oil
- 1 clove garlic, mashed
- 1½ heads kale, chopped
- ¼ teaspoon kosher salt
- 2 tablespoons toasted sesame seeds

Preparations

1. Prepare your oven preheated to 400°F.
2. Lightly and evenly grease baking sheet.
3. Pulse the Brazil nuts in a food processor until finely ground.
4. Put it in a small bowl and blend in breadcrumbs with Parmesan cheese.
5. Spread mustard evenly on tilapia fillets on your baking sheet.

6. Then, evenly spread Brazil nuts over tilapia.
7. Lightly spray with cooking spray.
8. Bake tilapia for about 8 to 10 minutes until cooked through.
9. While waiting, heat a large, stainless steel skillet with medium-high level.
10. Spray on sesame oil.
11. After about 15 seconds, add garlic.
12. Add chopped kale after 20 seconds.
13. Stirring frequently, let your kale cook about 7 to 8 minutes.
14. Toss in sesame seeds to combine.
15. Serve tilapia on a serving plate with the side of kale.

Red Pepper and Turkey Pasta

Ingredients
- 3 large red bell peppers
- 3 tbsp. of extra virgin olive oil
- 1 large onion (chopped)
- 2 tsp. garlic (minced)
- 2 tbsp. fresh oregano (chopped)
- 1 tbsp. of red wine vinegar
- 2 lbs. of ground turkey
- 2 lbs. of hot-cooked, protein-rich rigatoni

Preparations

1. Clean, cut and remove stem and seeds of peppers.
2. Coarsely chop peppers.
3. Heat oil in a large Dutch oven over medium heat.
4. Put in peppers with onions.
5. Cook until tender, usually takes 20 minutes.
6. Add garlic, cook for 5 minutes more.
7. Put mixture in a blender and make a smooth puree.
8. Reheat sauce on pan over medium-low heat.
9. Sprinkle the oregano and pour in vinegar.
10. Adjust seasonings for preferred taste.
11. In another skillet, sauté and cook ground turkey sprayed with a good vegetable cooking spray.
12. Mix cooked turkey into sauce and simmer.
13. After 15 to 20 minutes, serve turkey mix with the hot, cooked pasta.

Steamed Salmon with Lemon Scented Zucchini

Ingredients
- 1 onion, thinly sliced
- 1 lemon, thinly sliced
- 2 small zucchini, thinly sliced
- 1 cup white wine
- ½ cup of water
- 4 (6-ounce) salmon fillets
- ¼ tsp. of kosher salt
- ¼ tsp. of freshly ground pepper

Preparations
1. Place onion, lemon, zucchini, wine, and water in large Dutch oven.
2. Season the fish fillet evenly with pepper and salt.
3. Place a lightly greased steamer over the Dutch oven with the vegetable mixture at the bottom.
4. Put oven over medium-high heat.
5. Reduce heat when liquid begins to boil.
6. Carefully place the fish on steamer rack and cover.

7. Steam fish until cooked.
8. Serve salmon fillets over vegetables.
9. Top it with sliced olives.
10. Enjoy your meal.

Sweet Potato and Black Bean Burgers with Lime Mayonnaise

Ingredients
- ½ cup of reduced fat mayonnaise
- 1 lime
- ½ tsp of hot sauce
- Vegetable cooking spray
- 1 small onion (chopped)
- 1 jalapeno (minced)
- 2 tsp. of ground cumin
- 2 tsp .of garlic (minced)
- 2 cups of raw sweet potato (grated)
- 1 egg, lightly beaten
- 1 cup of plain breadcrumbs, divided
- Whole wheat hamburger buns
- 2 (14.5-ounce) cans black beans, drained, rinsed, and mashed

Mary Walsh

Preparations

1. Adjust your broiler to a medium-high heat.
2. Set oven racks with 4 to 5 inches distance from broiler.
3. In a small bowl, zest the lime and squeeze it as well.
4. Mix in mayonnaise and hot sauce; mix well to combine.
5. Set aside and refrigerate until serving.
6. Heat a large skillet over a medium-high heat.
7. Spray it evenly with cooking spray.
8. Put onions and cook until tender.
9. Add additional ingredients, the cumin, jalapeno, and garlic.
10. Cook for about 30 seconds.
11. Place mixture into a large bowl and blend in mashed black beans, sweet potato, breadcrumbs, and egg.
12. Stir and mix it well for even combination.
13. Form eight patties from the mixture.
14. Sprinkle patties with breadcrumbs.
15. On a baking sheet sprinkled well with cooking spray, and set your patties.

16. Broil it on oven for about 8 to 10 minutes per side.
17. Serve with toasted buns and lime mayonnaise.

Quinoa and Turkey Stuffed Peppers

Ingredients
- 1 cup of uncooked quinoa
- 2 cups of water
- ½ tsp of salt
- ½ cup of chicken stock
- ¼ cup of extra virgin olive oil
- 3 tbsp. of pecans (chopped and toasted)
- 2 tbsp. of chopped fresh parsley
- 2 tsp. of chopped fresh rosemary
- 3 red bell peppers
- ½ pound fully-cooked smoked turkey sausage, diced

Preparations
1. In a large saucepan, mix quinoa, stock, water, and salt together.
2. Bring mixture to a boil over a high heat.
3. Reduce heat, cover, and let it simmer for about 15 minutes.

4. Uncover when excess liquid has been absorbed.
5. Set aside for a while, about 5 minutes.
6. Put in sausage, pecans, oil, parsley, and rosemary.
7. Cut the peppers in half.
8. Scoop out the seeds and the membranes.
9. Cook peppers about 5 minutes in boiling water then drain.
10. Fill each half pepper with your quinoa mixture.
11. Place it on a lightly greased baking dish.
12. Bake for about 15 minutes on 350°F oven.

ABOUT THE AUTHOR

Mary Walsh (1974 - Present) was born in Sydney Australia. Her career in writing has flourished over the past years. She has focused her work on health, nutrition and diet and has helped a lot of women change their life styles.

Mary is also volunteer health worker and has travelled to many deprived areas of the world. Her goal is to reach out to as many individuals as possible as long as her breath allows.

Right now, Mary is writing from the underprivileged areas of the Asia Pacific, sharing her work and reaching out to educate children on proper health and hygiene.

Lightning Source UK Ltd.
Milton Keynes UK
UKHW02f1840290718
326466UK00020B/440/P